RESET YOUR HEALTH

How a diagnosis of silent reflux led
me to healing my gut, losing 10kg and
becoming a better version of myself.

Erin Beattie

Kindle Publishing

To my husband - Merlin, my children - Liam, Jacobie, Cooper and Aurora and my close family and friends - you know who you are.

You all stood by me as I struggled through bouts of poor health. You all supported my crazy hours of research, fed my horses when I couldn't, understood when I needed to leave gatherings prematurely and never questioned whatever new and wonderful food I was eating at any time.

You all are my strength, my reason why, and I will never forget the love and care you showed me throughout this entire healing journey.

*To Will - thanks for the encouragement.
Now you can read the book.*

CONTENTS

DISCLAIMER:

The information provided is based on my personal research and experiences, and what has worked for me. I am not a medical doctor or specialist. It is important to consult with a qualified healthcare professional or registered dietitian before making significant changes to your diet or lifestyle. Individual dietary needs and health conditions vary, and professional guidance can provide personalized recommendations tailored to your specific circumstances. This information is intended for educational purposes only and should not be construed as medical advice or a substitute for professional healthcare guidance.

I had always been health-conscious, so when I decided to embark on a week-long juice cleanse, I thought I was doing something good for my body. Little did I know, it would set off a chain of events that would leave both myself and Drs puzzled and seeking answers for months to come.

During the cleanse, I felt invigorated at first. The vibrant colours and fresh flavours seemed to promise a detoxified body and renewed energy. However, by the third day, I started experiencing discomfort in my stomach. Ignoring it, I pushed through, believing it was just my body adjusting to the cleanse. I focused a lot on fruits over vegetables, oranges, apples, strawberries, lime, lemon, grapefruit cucumber, carrots and beetroot were my go to foods to juice, little did I know the damage that the high citrus diet was causing to my digestive system.

As the days went on, the discomfort turned into persistent nausea, a tight feeling when breathing, fatigue and pains in the chest area. I thought perhaps it was a temporary reaction to the cleanse, but the symptoms persisted even after I resumed my normal diet. Concerned, I visited the ER first worried it was a problem with my heart and then I followed up my doctor, expecting a quick diagnosis and remedy.

What followed was a frustrating journey of medical appointments, tests, and conflicting opinions. Blood tests, stool tests, ultrasounds—all came back normal. Specialists were consulted, and still, no clear diagnosis emerged I was put on corticosteroid inhalers, H2RA blockers and long-acting COPD inhalers. Meanwhile, my symptoms persisted, affecting my daily life and leaving me increasingly anxious and worried for my family – what if I was terminally ill?

It wasn't until seven long months later, after a particularly thorough consultation with a new Dr, that the mystery began to unravel. The doctor listened carefully as I recounted my symptoms and medical history. He asked about any unusual sensations or patterns, prompting me to recall the persistent feeling of something stuck in my throat, especially after meals or when lying down as well as the constant post nasal drip and coughing.

Finally, a diagnosis: silent reflux, also known as laryngopharyngeal reflux (LPR). Unlike typical acid reflux, silent reflux often presents with throat symptoms rather than heartburn. The acidic stomach contents were creeping up into my throat, causing irritation and inflammation—a condition exacerbated by the acidity of the juices during my cleanse which was followed by a nasty bout of gastroenteritis a month later.

Relief washed over me, mingled with frustration at the long and arduous journey to this diagnosis. Treatment began with dietary changes, avoiding acidic foods and beverages, elevating the head of my bed, and taking medications - , proton pump inhibitors and nasal sprays - to reduce stomach acid production.

After researching the effects of proton pump inhibitors, I decide to remove them from my health plan and continue healing by utilising the correct way of eating and a few supplements known to help heal the digestive system.

Over time, as I adhered to the treatment plan, my symptoms gradually improved. The burning sensation and nausea subsided, and I regained my energy and optimism. Reflecting on the experience, I realized the importance of listening to my body and seeking thorough medical advice when symptoms persist.

The journey through silent reflux taught me patience, resilience, and the significance of comprehensive healthcare as well as my own due diligence when it came to researching natural alternatives. Though challenging, it ultimately led me to a path of healing and a deeper understanding of my own body's needs.

When I was diagnosed with silent reflux after months of uncertainty and discomfort, I was determined to find a natural way to heal. Armed with determination and a thirst for knowledge, I delved into hours of research, scouring articles, forums, and medical journals for information on dietary protocols that could alleviate my symptoms.

The first protocol I stumbled upon emphasized alkaline foods—leafy greens, non-citrus fruits, and lean proteins. The rationale was simple: reducing acidity in the diet could help neutralize stomach acid and ease the inflammation in my throat. Excitedly, I stocked my fridge with kale, spinach, and cucumbers, and swapped out my morning coffee for herbal tea.

In the initial weeks, I noticed some improvement. The burning sensation in my throat lessened, and the feeling of something stuck began to fade. Encouraged by these results but still seeking more comprehensive relief, I continued my quest.

Next, I came across a low-acid diet plan, which focused on avoiding not just highly acidic foods like tomatoes and citrus fruits but also acidic beverages and processed foods. I meticulously crafted meal plans, steering clear of triggers identified in the diet guidelines. Breakfasts became oatmeal with almond milk, lunches consisted of grilled chicken and steamed vegetables, and dinners were hearty yet gentle on my stomach.

This approach brought further relief. Days turned into weeks, and my symptoms continued to diminish. Yet, I remained curious about other potential solutions. That's when I stumbled upon a third dietary approach: the Carnivore diet. Emphasizing organic meat, eggs and dairy, this diet boasted anti-inflammatory benefits and a focus on resetting your health.

Intrigued, I decided to blend elements from all three protocols. After 4 weeks of doing a carnivore reset, I gradually introduced a keto/wholefood hybrid diet. I started my mornings with a green smoothie—kale, banana, oats and almond milk—to alkalize and soothe. For lunch salad with mixed greens, grilled chicken, avocado, and a drizzle of extra virgin olive oil. Dinners were light yet satisfying, often featuring baked fish with quinoa and roasted vegetables. Snacks were homemade beef jerky, eggs or greek yoghurt. I also incorporated 2 glasses of filmjolk a day (the Swedish version of fermented milk)

As I adopted this hybrid approach, I noticed a remarkable improvement in my overall well-being. The burning sensation disappeared completely, and the nagging feeling of discomfort in my throat subsided. With each passing day, I felt more energized and optimistic about my journey toward healing.

Reflecting on my experience, I realized that healing isn't always a linear path but rather a personalized journey of discovery and adaptation. By integrating the best elements of various dietary protocols and listening closely to my body's responses, I found a sustainable way to manage and eventually overcome silent reflux.

Today, armed with newfound knowledge and a deeper connection to my body's needs, I continue to prioritize balanced eating and mindful living. My journey with silent reflux taught me resilience, patience, and the power of self-care—a lesson I carry with me as I navigate life's challenges with renewed vigour and gratitude.

In the midst of bustling days and savory meals, I found myself grappling with a persistent discomfort—a burning sensation that crept up my throat after meals, accompanied by bloating and occasional regurgitation. It wasn't until I sought answers from healthcare professionals that I discovered the culprit behind my symptoms: acid reflux.

Armed with this diagnosis, I embarked on a journey to reclaim digestive comfort by identifying and navigating foods that triggered reflux—a journey that required mindfulness and a newfound awareness of the impact of dietary choices on my well-being.

Among the foods to avoid with reflux, acidic and spicy fare topped the list. Tangy citrus fruits, tomatoes, and their derivatives like marinara sauce proved to be potent triggers, exacerbating the acid in my stomach and leading to discomfort. Spicy dishes, once a source of culinary excitement, now posed a challenge as they stimulated acid production and intensified reflux symptoms.

Carbonated beverages, with their bubbly effervescence, also made the list of offenders. The carbon dioxide gas in sodas and sparkling waters expanded in my stomach, causing bloating and increasing pressure that pushed stomach acid upwards towards the oesophagus—a recipe for reflux disaster.

Chocolate, a beloved indulgence, emerged as a surprising culprit due to its combination of fat and caffeine, both of which can relax the lower oesophageal sphincter (LES) and allow acid to reflux into the oesophagus more easily. Alongside chocolate, fried and fatty foods posed a similar risk, as their high fat content delayed stomach emptying and prolonged the presence of food in the stomach—heightening the likelihood of reflux.

Caffeine, found not only in coffee but also in tea, energy

drinks, and some medications, proved challenging to navigate. Its stimulant effect on gastric acid production and potential to relax the LES made it a trigger for reflux symptoms, prompting me to explore decaffeinated alternatives or limit intake to support digestive comfort.

Armed with this knowledge, I embarked on a journey of culinary exploration, discovering delicious alternatives and mindful substitutes that supported my quest for reflux relief. I embraced lean proteins, whole grains, and fiber-rich fruits and vegetables —choosing foods that nourished my body without triggering discomfort.

Through mindful choices and a commitment to listening to my body's signals, I found relief from reflux symptoms and regained a sense of balance in my dietary habits. Each meal became an opportunity to support digestive health, fostering a deeper connection to the nourishing power of food and its impact on my well-being.

Reflecting on my journey with foods to avoid with reflux, I realized the importance of personalized dietary strategies in managing digestive disorders. By navigating triggers and embracing supportive foods, I reclaimed control over my health and embarked on a path to sustainable comfort and vitality—a journey that continues to inspire me to prioritize mindful eating and holistic well-being in every aspect of life.

In the midst of hectic schedules and dietary uncertainties, I found myself at a crossroads—a desire for renewed health and vitality that propelled me towards a transformative journey. Faced with excess weight and persistent digestive discomfort, I embarked on a path guided by intuition, listening to my body's cues and embracing a holistic approach to wellness centred on healing the gut and embracing reflux-friendly foods.

My journey began with a pivotal realization—that my body was speaking to me through symptoms like acid reflux, bloating, and occasional discomfort. Armed with this awareness, I sought guidance from healthcare professionals who emphasized the interconnectedness of gut health and overall well-being.

Inspired by insights into the gut's pivotal role in digestion, immunity, and metabolism, I adopted a strategy focused on healing and nourishing my gut. I prioritized whole, unprocessed foods that supported digestive health—opting for lean proteins like chicken and fish, fibre-rich vegetables, and complex carbohydrates such as quinoa and sweet potatoes. These choices not only provided essential nutrients but also promoted satiety and stable energy levels throughout the day.

Crucially, I identified and avoided trigger foods that exacerbated reflux symptoms—steering clear of acidic fruits, spicy dishes, caffeine, and fatty foods that had once contributed to digestive discomfort. Instead, I embraced alkaline alternatives and soothing herbal teas that calmed inflammation and supported a balanced pH environment in my stomach.

Mindful eating became a cornerstone of my daily routine. I savoured each bite, tuning into sensations of hunger and fullness, and honouring my body's signals. Portion control and balanced meals ensured I maintained steady progress towards my weight loss goals, while also nurturing a positive relationship with food based on nourishment and respect for my body's needs.

As weeks passed, the transformative effects of my dietary adjustments became evident. The excess weight began to melt away, revealing a leaner, more energetic version of myself. I experienced increased vitality and mental clarity—a testament to the healing power of supporting gut health and making conscious dietary choices.

Beyond physical changes, I discovered a profound sense of empowerment and self-discovery. By listening to my body and embracing a holistic approach to health, I not only shed pounds but also cultivated resilience and a deeper understanding of the intricate balance between nutrition, digestion, and overall well-being.

Reflecting on my journey to losing 10kg in 8 weeks by healing my gut and embracing reflux-friendly foods, I realized that sustainable health and vitality are attainable through mindful choices and a commitment to holistic wellness. Each step was a testament to the transformative power of listening to my body's wisdom and prioritising self-care—a journey that continues to inspire me to embrace a balanced lifestyle rooted in nourishment, healing, and lifelong well-being.

When people think of trigger foods, they think of foods that affect them emotionally – foods they turn to for comfort or that bring them joy, foods that can bring up memories or ones they associate with certain people or place. For reflux, trigger foods are those that cause any type of symptom or discomfort.

Citrus, spices, caffeine, alcohol, eggs – anything that you ingest that causes discomfort needs to be eliminated until your body has healed and your microbiome is balanced. For me, my main trigger foods were carbonated drinks, caffeine, nightshades, citrus, oils, bread and mint. I even had to find mint free toothpaste. After 3visits to hospital with chest pains after drinking fizzy drink, I will now have carbonated drinks ingrained in my brain as a strict no go drink for the rest of my life.

Armed with a determination to take charge of my health, I started keeping a detailed food diary. Every meal and snack, along with the time and any symptoms I experienced afterward, were meticulously recorded. Over time, patterns began to emerge. I noticed that certain foods consistently triggered my reflux symptoms—spicy foods, citrus fruits, chocolate, and fried dishes were among the culprits.

With the help of my food diary, I gradually eliminated or reduced my intake of the identified trigger foods. Instead, I focused on incorporating more whole foods into my diet—lean proteins, vegetables, fruits with low acidity, whole grains, and healthy fats. It wasn't always easy, especially when social events or cravings tempted me to indulge in my old favourites. However, the relief from reduced reflux symptoms provided the motivation I needed to stay on track.

As I made these dietary changes to manage my reflux, I began to notice something unexpected—I was losing weight.

The combination of eliminating trigger foods and focusing on healthier options naturally led to a reduction in calorie intake. I wasn't following a strict diet or counting calories; instead, I was simply making choices that supported both my digestive health and my overall well-being.

As months passed, my efforts started to pay off. Not only did my reflux symptoms become less frequent and less severe, but I also shed excess pounds. My energy levels improved, and I felt more confident and in control of my health. What had started as a quest to alleviate discomfort had evolved into a transformative journey toward a healthier lifestyle.

Today, I continue to prioritize my health by maintaining a balanced diet that supports digestive health and overall wellness. I've learned to listen to my body and recognize its signals, whether it's a craving for nutrient-rich foods or a reminder to stay hydrated. I still enjoy occasional treats in moderation, knowing that balance is key to long-term success.

When my battle with silent reflux escalated, I sought relief through conventional means. My doctor prescribed proton pump inhibitors (PPIs) and histamine-2 receptor antagonists (H2RAs) with assurances of symptom relief and healing. Initially, these medications seemed like a lifeline, offering respite from the persistent discomfort and acid reflux.

However, as weeks turned into months, I started noticing subtle changes in my health. Despite the initial relief, I began experiencing new symptoms—fatigue, headaches, and digestive issues. Alarmed, I consulted my doctor, who assured me these were unrelated or minor side effects.

Determined to understand the root cause, I delved into research about PPIs and H2RAs. What I discovered was eye-opening and concerning. PPIs, while effective at reducing stomach acid, can disrupt the natural balance of gut flora, leading to digestive issues like diarrhoea, bloating, and nutrient deficiencies. Long-term use has been associated with increased risks of osteoporosis, kidney disease, and even cognitive decline.

Similarly, H2RAs, though considered less potent than PPIs, can also alter gut microbiota and potentially contribute to nutrient malabsorption over time. Moreover, both classes of medications can lead to dependency, where the body becomes accustomed to their effects, necessitating higher doses or prolonged use for continued relief.

Feeling conflicted and worried about the long-term consequences, I decided to explore alternative approaches to managing my silent reflux. With guidance from a holistic practitioner, I gradually weaned off PPIs and H2RAs under careful supervision. Embracing natural remedies and lifestyle modifications became my new focus.

I turned to dietary changes, adopting a low-acid diet rich in whole grains, fruits, and vegetables. I incorporated probiotics and digestive enzymes to support gut health and optimize digestion. Stress management techniques such as yoga and meditation helped reduce triggers for reflux episodes.

As I implemented these changes, I noticed a gradual improvement in my symptoms. The burning sensation in my throat lessened, and I regained energy and clarity of mind. Unlike the temporary relief provided by medications, these holistic approaches addressed the underlying factors contributing to my silent reflux.

Reflecting on my journey, I realized the importance of informed choices and personalized care in managing health conditions. While PPIs and H2RAs can offer immediate relief, their potential risks underscore the need for caution and exploration of alternative therapies. My experience taught me to prioritize holistic health practices that promote balance and sustainability, empowering me to reclaim control of my well-being without compromising long-term health.

In the intricate tapestry of the human body, there exists a vibrant ecosystem that plays a profound role in our overall health and well-being—the gut microbiome. Like a bustling city teeming with diverse inhabitants, this microscopic community of bacteria, fungi, viruses, and other microorganisms inhabits our gastrointestinal tract, influencing everything from digestion to immune function and even mental health.

My journey into understanding the significance of the gut microbiome began with a curiosity sparked by persistent health issues. For years, I struggled with digestive discomfort, recurring infections, and fluctuating energy levels. Despite seeking conventional treatments, the root causes remained elusive until I stumbled upon the concept of the gut microbiome through extensive research and discussions with healthcare professionals.

I learned that the gut microbiome is not just a passive bystander in our digestive system but a dynamic entity that interacts closely with our bodies. It plays a crucial role in breaking down food, extracting nutrients, and producing essential vitamins like B12 and K. Moreover, these microbial communities communicate with our immune system, helping to regulate inflammation and defend against pathogens.

Beyond its digestive functions, the gut microbiome influences our mental health and brain function through the gut-brain axis—a bidirectional communication pathway between the gut and the central nervous system. Emerging research suggests that disruptions in the gut microbiome composition may contribute to conditions such as anxiety, depression, and even neurological disorders.

As I delved deeper into nurturing my gut health, I adopted

strategies to support a diverse and balanced microbiome. I focused on incorporating fibre-rich foods like fruits, vegetables, and whole grains, which serve as prebiotics—nutrients that fuel the growth of beneficial gut bacteria. Probiotic-rich foods like yogurt, kefir, and fermented vegetables became staples, introducing beneficial bacteria directly into my gut.

I also paid attention to lifestyle factors that impact the gut microbiome, such as stress management, adequate sleep, and regular physical activity. These practices helped create an environment conducive to a thriving microbial community, promoting optimal digestion, immune function, and overall vitality.

Over time, as I nurtured my gut microbiome with mindful choices and a holistic approach to health, I began to experience profound improvements. Digestive discomfort eased, recurrent infections became less frequent, and my energy levels stabilized. More importantly, I gained a deeper appreciation for the interconnectedness of our body's systems and the pivotal role of the gut microbiome in maintaining balance and resilience.

Reflecting on my journey, I realized that cultivating a healthy gut microbiome is not just about digestive health but a cornerstone of overall well-being. By nourishing this intricate ecosystem within us, we empower our bodies to thrive, supporting longevity and vitality in every aspect of life. My journey with the gut microbiome continues to inspire me to prioritize gut health as a foundation for holistic wellness—a journey that unfolds with each mindful choice and fosters a deeper connection to the remarkable symbiosis within us.

In the vibrant tapestry of my life, I never truly grasped the impact of what I ate until a series of health challenges prompted me to delve deeper into the world of inflammatory foods and their profound effects on the body. It began with subtle signals—a lingering fatigue, occasional joint pain, and digestive discomfort that seemed to ebb and flow without clear cause.

Like many, I cherished the convenience and indulgence of modern diets, often reaching for processed foods, sugary treats, and refined carbohydrates without much thought. These culinary delights, while satisfying in the moment, concealed a hidden truth—they were fuelling an inflammatory response within my body.

Curiosity led me down a path of exploration, guided by insights from healthcare professionals and extensive research. I discovered that certain foods—such as refined sugars, processed meats, trans fats, and excessive alcohol—can trigger inflammation in the body. This inflammatory response is mediated by the immune system, which perceives these substances as foreign invaders and mounts a defence.

Inflammation, when acute, is a natural and necessary response that helps the body heal from injuries and infections. However, chronic inflammation, driven by prolonged exposure to inflammatory foods and other lifestyle factors, can wreak havoc on health. It is linked to a myriad of conditions including cardiovascular disease, diabetes, autoimmune disorders, and even cancer.

Armed with this knowledge, I embarked on a journey to reclaim my health by adopting an anti-inflammatory diet. I focused on whole, nutrient-dense foods such as leafy greens, colourful fruits and vegetables, fatty fish rich in omega-3 fatty acids, nuts, seeds, and olive oil. These foods are known for their anti-inflammatory properties, helping to quench the fire of inflammation within.

As I made these dietary adjustments, I began to notice profound changes in my well-being. The nagging fatigue lifted, joint pain diminished, and digestive issues became less frequent. More importantly, I felt a renewed sense of vitality and resilience—a testament to the transformative power of nourishing my body with foods that support rather than sabotage its natural balance.

Beyond dietary changes, I embraced holistic practices to further reduce inflammation and support overall health. Regular physical activity, stress management techniques like yoga and meditation, and adequate sleep became integral parts of my daily routine. These lifestyle adjustments complemented my dietary choices, creating a holistic approach to healing and well-being.

Reflecting on my journey with inflammatory foods and the body's response, I gained a deeper appreciation for the profound connection between diet and health. By honouring my body's innate wisdom and making conscious choices to reduce inflammation, I not only restored balance but also unlocked a newfound vitality and vitality in every aspect of my life

In the sweltering heat of summer, there's nothing quite like the refreshing relief of an ice-cold drink or a scoop of frozen dessert. For years, I indulged in these icy pleasures without a second thought—until my digestive system began to rebel, prompting me to reconsider the consequences of my chilly habits.

Whilst delving into research to help cure my silent reflux, I learned that consuming ice-cold substances can shock the digestive system, slowing down the natural process of digestion. This delay can lead to bloating as food sits longer in the stomach, struggling to break down properly.

Moreover, the extreme temperature contrast—going from hot weather outside to a sudden intake of cold—can disrupt the delicate balance of enzymes and acids required for efficient digestion. This imbalance can exacerbate symptoms of acid reflux or gastritis, making the discomfort more pronounced and persistent.

As I reflected on my dietary habits, I realized that my love for cold treats had unwittingly contributed to my digestive woes. The habit of consuming icy beverages with meals or enjoying chilled desserts had become ingrained in my routine, overshadowing the potential consequences for my gut health.

Determined to restore harmony to my digestive system, I embarked on a journey of mindful eating. I gradually replaced ice-cold drinks with room temperature alternatives, allowing my body to digest fluids more smoothly. I opted for warm herbal teas and infused waters to stay hydrated without shocking my system.

Similarly, I adjusted my approach to meals, opting for warm or at least not overly chilled foods whenever possible. This shift not only eased the discomfort but also encouraged a deeper connection with the natural rhythms of my body's digestion.

Over time, as I embraced these changes, I noticed a significant improvement in my digestive health. The bloating and cramps subsided, replaced by a sense of ease and vitality. I realized that by respecting the needs of my digestive system and choosing foods and beverages thoughtfully, I could support its optimal function and overall well-being.

My journey with the chilling effects on digestive health taught me an invaluable lesson: balance and moderation are key. While occasional indulgence in cold treats is enjoyable, understanding their impact and making conscious choices can make a profound difference in maintaining digestive harmony. By listening to my body and prioritizing its needs, I discovered a path to greater comfort and vitality—one warm sip at a time.

In the bustling city where I live, carbonated beverages were ubiquitous. From soda fountains on street corners to shelves packed with fizzy drinks in every convenience store, they seemed like a refreshing and harmless indulgence. Little did I know, these bubbly concoctions would soon reveal their hidden impact on my body.

It all began innocently enough—a casual drink with friends at a local diner. The satisfying hiss of carbonation and the cool rush of bubbles down my throat offered instant gratification on a hot summer day. Yet, beneath the surface, my body was silently reacting.

As weeks turned into months of undiagnosed silent reflux, I started noting more and more discomfort after drinking a fizzy drink. Initially, it was the occasional bloating or feeling uncomfortably full after drinking. Dismissing these as minor inconveniences, I continued to enjoy my favourite carbonated beverages without much thought.

However, the symptoms escalated. Persistent bloating turned into frequent bouts of gas and discomfort. I began experiencing chest pain and heaviness that let to visits to the emergency department at my local hospital. Alarmed by these developments, I sought advice from a healthcare professional who shed light on the detrimental effects of carbonated beverages.

I learned that the carbon dioxide gas present in these drinks can expand in the stomach, leading to bloating and distension. This bloating can exacerbate conditions like irritable bowel syndrome (IBS) and contribute to abdominal discomfort as well as an unbalanced gut microbiome.

Furthermore, the acidity of many carbonated beverages—

especially colas—can erode tooth enamel over time, increasing the risk of dental cavities and tooth decay. The high sugar content in sodas can also contribute to weight gain and metabolic disorders when consumed regularly.

Armed with this newfound knowledge, I made a conscious decision to reduce my intake of carbonated beverages. I gradually replaced sodas with healthier alternatives like water infused with fresh fruits or herbal teas. The transition wasn't easy, as the allure of fizz and flavour remained strong, but my commitment to improving my health prevailed.

As weeks passed, I began to notice positive changes. The bloating and discomfort subsided, and my digestion felt more settled and balanced. I no longer experienced the sharp pangs of acid reflux after meals, and my energy levels stabilized without the highs and crashes induced by sugary sodas.

Reflecting on my journey with carbonated beverages, I realized that moderation and awareness are crucial. While the occasional fizzy drink can be a treat, understanding its potential effects on the body and making informed choices is essential for long-term health and well-being. By listening to my body's signals and prioritizing its needs, I discovered a path to greater vitality and resilience—a journey that continues to inspire mindful choices in every sip.

For many years, my mornings began with the comforting ritual of a steaming cup of coffee and a square of rich, dark chocolate. These indulgences seemed innocuous—a source of pleasure and a boost of energy to kickstart my day. However, beneath their allure lay a journey of discovery into their complex effects on my digestive system.

The love affair with caffeine began after high school, where working 3 jobs and long hours made coffee a constant companion. The energizing effects were undeniable; helping me power through long hours with renewed focus. Yet, as my dependence on caffeine grew, so did the toll on my digestive health.

I started experiencing symptoms like acid reflux and heartburn, especially after my morning coffee. The acidic nature of coffee, coupled with its stimulating effect on gastric acid production, contributed to discomfort and a persistent burning sensation in my chest. Concerned, I spent many hours researching the impact of caffeine on digestive function.

I learned that caffeine can relax the lower oesophageal sphincter (LES), the muscle that normally prevents stomach acid from flowing back into the oesophagus. This relaxation can lead to acid reflux and exacerbate symptoms in individuals prone to digestive disorders like gastroesophageal reflux disease (GERD).

Determined to alleviate my symptoms, I gradually reduced my coffee intake and explored alternatives like green tea, which has lower caffeine content and is generally less acidic. The transition wasn't easy, as coffee had become intertwined with my daily routine and social interactions. Yet, with perseverance and mindful choices, I began to notice improvements in my digestive comfort.

However, my journey didn't end with caffeine alone. I soon discovered that chocolate, another beloved indulgence, could also trigger digestive distress. Dark chocolate, in particular, contains compounds like theobromine and caffeine that can stimulate the production of stomach acid and relax the LES, similar to coffee.

As much as I enjoyed the rich flavour and antioxidant benefits of dark chocolate, I had to acknowledge its potential impact on my digestive system. Consuming chocolate in moderation became key, and I opted for ceremonial cocoa or enjoyed it as an occasional treat rather than a daily habit.

Through mindful experimentation and a deeper understanding of how caffeine and chocolate affect my body, I found a balanced approach that supports digestive harmony. Today, I start my mornings with a cup of warm water, savouring the moments of quiet reflection without the discomfort of acid reflux. Occasional indulgences in chocolate are enjoyed consciously, with an awareness of their potential effects and a commitment to overall well-being.

My journey with caffeine and chocolate taught me valuable lessons about listening to my body's signals and making informed choices that prioritize digestive health. By embracing moderation and mindfulness in my dietary habits, I discovered a path to greater comfort, vitality, and enjoyment of life's simple pleasures —a journey that continues to evolve with each mindful sip and bite.

Growing up in a country town, social gatherings often revolved around the clinking of glasses and the cheers of celebratory toasts. For years, I embraced the convivial atmosphere of bars and parties, where alcohol flowed freely and seemed an integral part of social interaction. Yet, beneath the surface of these festive moments lay a journey of discovery into the profound effects of alcohol on gut health.

Like many, my relationship with alcohol began casually—a drink here and there to unwind after a long day or to toast a special occasion. The initial effects were immediate and seemingly harmless—a sense of relaxation and euphoria that temporarily lifted my spirits. However, as time went on, I started noticing subtle changes in my well-being, particularly in my digestive comfort.

The first signs were mild—a slight queasiness after a night of indulgence or occasional bloating. Dismissing these as transient inconveniences, I continued to partake in social drinking without much concern. Yet, as my consumption increased during social events and stressful periods, the symptoms intensified.

I began experiencing more discomfort and concerning symptoms, even after only drinking ne alcoholic beverage. The acidic nature of alcohol can irritate the lining of the stomach and oesophagus, leading to inflammation and discomfort. This irritation can weaken the lower oesophageal sphincter (LES), allowing stomach acid to reflux into the oesophagus more easily—a condition known as gastroesophageal reflux disease (GERD).

As I delved into the rabbit warren of information surrounding silent reflux, I learned that alcohol can disrupt the balance of beneficial bacteria in the gut microbiome, potentially contributing to dysbiosis—a condition characterized by an imbalance of gut flora linked to digestive disorders and immune system dysfunction.

Moreover, alcohol can impair the function of the intestinal barrier, often referred to as "leaky gut syndrome." This condition allows toxins, bacteria, and undigested food particles to pass through the intestinal lining into the bloodstream, triggering inflammation and immune responses throughout the body.

Determined to prioritise my gut health, I embarked on a journey of mindful drinking and moderation. I reduced my alcohol intake, opting for lighter options like wine or beer on occasion and savouring each glass slowly. I also explored non-alcoholic alternatives during social gatherings, focusing on the company and conversation rather than the contents of my glass.

As I made these adjustments, I noticed a significant improvement in my digestive comfort and overall well-being. The acid reflux and bloating subsided, replaced by a sense of clarity and vitality. Embracing this newfound balance, I realized the profound impact of alcohol on gut health and the importance of making informed choices to support digestive harmony.

Reflecting on my journey with alcohol, I discovered that moderation and mindfulness are essential. By listening to my body's signals and respecting its limits, I found a path to greater digestive comfort and overall vitality—a journey that continues to inspire me to prioritize holistic health practices in every aspect of life.

In the bustling rhythm of modern life, where convenience often dictates our dietary choices, I discovered a profound truth about the transformative power of whole foods. It was a realisation born from personal experience—a journey of rediscovering health and vitality through the simplicity and wholesomeness of nature's bounty.

My story begins with a series of health challenges—persistent fatigue, digestive discomfort, and fluctuating energy levels— later diagnosed as silent reflux that prompted a deeper exploration into the relationship between food and well-being. Frustrated by temporary fixes and quick fixes that failed to address the root causes, I turned to whole foods as a holistic approach to nourishing my body and soul.

Whole foods, by definition, are unprocessed or minimally processed foods that retain their natural nutrients and beneficial compounds. They encompass a vibrant spectrum of fruits, vegetables, whole grains, nuts, seeds, legumes, and lean proteins— all essential components of a balanced diet that supports optimal health.

Embracing the concept of whole foods meant prioritizing nutrient density over calorie count, choosing foods that provide essential vitamins, minerals, antioxidants, and fibre in their natural form. It meant savouring the crisp sweetness of an apple, the earthy richness of whole grains, and the satisfying crunch of nuts and seeds—each bite a celebration of nourishment and vitality.

As I integrated more whole foods into my daily meals, I began to notice profound changes in my health and well-being. The persistent fatigue lifted, replaced by sustained energy and mental clarity. Digestive discomfort diminished as my gut responded to the fibre-rich foods that supported healthy digestion and nutrient absorption.

Beyond physical improvements, I discovered a deeper connection to the earth's bounty and the interconnectedness of food, body, and environment. Whole foods became a cornerstone of my culinary repertoire, inspiring creativity in the kitchen and a sense of mindfulness in every meal preparation.

Moreover, I learned that whole foods are not just about nutrition—they are about honouring the integrity of natural ingredients and supporting sustainable food practices that respect the planet. By choosing whole foods, I embraced a lifestyle that aligned with my values of health, sustainability, and holistic well-being.

Reflecting on my journey with whole foods, I realized their transformative power extends beyond the dinner plate. They nourish not only the body but also the soul, fostering a profound sense of vitality, connection, and gratitude for the abundance of nature's gifts. My journey continues to inspire me to prioritize whole foods as a foundation for lifelong health and wellness—a journey that celebrates the simplicity and richness of eating well for life.

In a world of culinary complexity and endless food choices, I embarked on a journey that celebrated the beauty and nourishment found in simplicity—the importance of eating foods with only one ingredient, or combining each individual ingredient mindfully to create wholesome recipes that honour their essence.

It all began with a realization sparked by a desire for clarity and vitality in my daily diet. Faced with shelves lined with packaged goods boasting exotic flavours and convenience, I yearned for a return to basics—a return to foods that spoke for themselves in their natural state.

The concept was straightforward yet profound: foods with only one ingredient—whether it be an apple picked from a nearby orchard, a handful of nuts gathered from the earth, or a cut of grass-fed beef from a local farm—held a purity and authenticity that resonated deeply with me.

I embraced the simplicity of single ingredients as a guiding principle in my culinary choices. Each meal became a canvas where I celebrated the intrinsic flavours and nutritional richness of whole foods. Fresh fruits and vegetables, minimally processed grains, and lean proteins formed the foundation of my plate, each ingredient chosen for its quality and nourishing properties.

By focusing on foods with one ingredient, I discovered a newfound appreciation for their innate goodness. Whole fruits and vegetables delivered a spectrum of vitamins, minerals, and antioxidants that supported my immune system and overall vitality. Nuts and seeds provided essential fats and proteins, while whole grains offered sustained energy and fiber for digestive health.

Moreover, I learned the art of mindful combination—pairing individual ingredients thoughtfully to create recipes that celebrated their unique flavours and textures. Simple salads burst with vibrant colours and crisp freshness, while hearty soups simmered with depth and warmth from wholesome ingredients. Each dish became a testament to the synergy of real foods, united in harmony to nourish body and soul.

As I embraced the importance of eating foods with only one ingredient or combining them mindfully, I noticed transformative changes in my well-being. Digestive discomfort faded, replaced by a sense of balance and ease. Energy levels stabilized, and mental clarity sharpened—a reflection of the nourishing power found in nature's bounty.

Beyond the physical benefits, I discovered a deeper connection to the origins of my food and a reverence for the farmers and producers who cultivated these gifts of the earth. Each ingredient carried a story—a story of growth, harvest, and the journey from farm to table—a narrative that enriched my culinary experience and deepened my appreciation for the interconnectedness of food and community.

Reflecting on my journey with foods of one ingredient, I realized their profound impact on my health, happiness, and connection to the natural world. By honoring the simplicity and purity of real food, I cultivated a lifestyle that prioritizes nourishment, sustainability, and holistic well-being—a journey that continues to inspire me to embrace the essence of each ingredient and celebrate the richness of eating well.

In the depths of internet research, I discovered a timeless secret to health and vitality—fermented foods. This revelation emerged from a journey of exploration into the intricate relationship between diet and gut health, guided by the wisdom passed down through generations.

Fermented foods, revered for their probiotic-rich properties, became a cornerstone of my quest to nourish and heal my gut. The journey began with fermented dairy—like yogurt and kefir —whose tangy flavours and creamy textures offered a delightful departure from conventional dietary norms. These cultured delights, brimming with beneficial bacteria such as lactobacilli and bifidobacteria, held the key to restoring balance within my digestive system.

As I embraced fermented dairy into my daily routine, I noticed subtle shifts in my well-being. Digestive discomfort, which had once punctuated my meals with unease, began to ease. Bloating diminished, and regularity became a welcome norm. It was as if my gut was rejoicing in the influx of probiotic reinforcements, fostering an environment where beneficial bacteria could flourish and thrive.

Inspired by the transformative effects of fermented dairy, I expanded my culinary horizons to include an array of fermented foods—from sauerkraut and kimchi to miso and tempeh. Each ferment offered a unique blend of flavours and textures, enriched by the fermentation process that unlocked their nutritional potential.

Fermented foods, I learned, not only enhance digestion but also support immune function, improve nutrient absorption, and contribute to overall well-being. The fermentation process breaks down complex carbohydrates and proteins into more easily digestible forms, while also producing vitamins, enzymes, and short-chain fatty acids that nourish the gut lining and support a healthy microbial balance.

As I continued to incorporate fermented foods into my diet, I experienced a deeper connection to the ancient wisdom of nourishing foods and their profound impact on holistic health. Beyond their nutritional benefits, fermented foods became a celebration of cultural heritage and a testament to the artistry of culinary traditions passed down through generations.

Moreover, I discovered that fermenting foods at home—an act of patience and care—fostered a deeper appreciation for the alchemy of transformation that occurs within each jar or crock. It connected me to the rhythms of nature and the seasons, reminding me of the symbiotic relationship between humans and the microbial world that sustains us.

Reflecting on my journey with fermented foods, I realised their power extends far beyond the realm of nutrition—they embody a holistic approach to health that honours the interconnectedness of body, mind, and spirit. By embracing fermented foods, I cultivated a flourishing ecosystem within my gut—a vibrant community of beneficial bacteria that supports resilience, vitality, and a deep sense of well-being.

In the quest for better digestion and overall well-being, one simple yet profoundly effective habit emerged as a game-changer for me: drinking warm water with every meal. This practice, rooted in ancient traditions across various cultures, has stood the test of time for good reason—it supports and enhances our digestive system in ways we may not fully appreciate in our modern, fast-paced lives.

Digestion begins the moment food enters our mouth and continues through a complex process involving enzymes, acids, and gut microbiota. One crucial element in this process is temperature. Our stomach and intestines function optimally within a certain temperature range, ideally around 98.6°F (37°C). When we consume cold beverages or food, especially during meals, we risk chilling these vital organs, potentially slowing down digestion and compromising nutrient absorption.

Warm water helps to stimulate the production of digestive enzymes and gastric juices. These enzymes break down food more efficiently, aiding in the absorption of nutrients and reducing the likelihood of indigestion or bloating. Drinking warm water with meals can promote smoother muscle contractions in the stomach and intestines, facilitating the movement of food through the digestive tract. This can alleviate constipation and promote regularity.

Warm water can help to improve blood circulation to the digestive organs. This increased blood flow enhances their efficiency in breaking down food and absorbing nutrients, contributing to overall digestive health. For those prone to acidity or heartburn, warm water can provide relief by neutralizing excess stomach acid and soothing the lining of the stomach.

Proper hydration is essential for optimal digestion. While water at any temperature hydrates, warm water is often more palatable during meals and encourages mindful drinking, ensuring we meet our daily hydration needs.

Making the switch to drinking warm water with meals is a simple yet powerful adjustment that can yield significant benefits over time. Here are practical tips to incorporate this habit into your daily routine. Aim to drink water around 15-30 minutes before meals to prime your digestive system, and continue during and after meals to support ongoing digestion.

In the pursuit of optimal digestion and overall well-being, the choice to drink warm water with every meal is a small yet impactful step. By supporting digestive enzyme activity, promoting smoother muscle contractions, and enhancing nutrient absorption, warm water can significantly contribute to a healthier digestive system. This ancient practice not only aligns with cultural wisdom but also resonates with modern scientific understanding of digestive physiology. Embrace this simple habit and experience the transformative benefits it brings to your daily life.

In my quest for a reflux friendly alternative to wheat, my research uncovered seeds and grains that I had never cooked with before. These add variety to my diet along with the following health benefits.

1. Chia Seeds: Chia seeds are very low in net carbs, high in fibre, and rich in healthy fats. Chia seeds contain omega-3 fatty acids, which have potent anti-inflammatory properties. They also provide antioxidants like quercetin, which can help reduce inflammation.

2. Flaxseeds: Flaxseeds are low in net carbs and high in fibre, making them suitable for a ketogenic diet. Flaxseeds are rich in alpha-linolenic acid (ALA), a type of omega-3 fatty acid known for its anti-inflammatory effects. They also contain lignans, which have antioxidant properties.

3. Hemp Seeds: Hemp seeds are low in net carbs and high in protein and healthy fats. Hemp seeds contain a balanced ratio of omega-6 to omega-3 fatty acids, which can help reduce inflammation in the body. They also provide gamma-linolenic acid (GLA), another anti-inflammatory fatty acid.

4. Quinoa (in moderation): Quinoa is higher in carbs compared to chia, flax, and hemp seeds but can still be included in small amounts on a ketogenic diet. Quinoa contains antioxidants such as quercetin and kaempferol, which have anti-inflammatory properties. It also provides fibre and plant-based protein, contributing to its overall health benefits.

By incorporating these keto-friendly and anti-inflammatory grains and seeds into your diet in appropriate portions, you can enjoy their nutritional benefits while supporting your ketogenic and overall health goals. As always, consult with a healthcare professional or registered dietitian to tailor your diet to your individual needs and health conditions.

Oats are often considered beneficial for their potential anti-inflammatory properties, especially due to certain compounds they contain. While oats themselves are not typically considered part of a strict ketogenic diet due to their carbohydrate content, they can still be included in moderation in a low-carb or balanced diet for their potential health benefits, including anti-inflammatory effects. Here's a look at how oats can contribute to reducing inflammation:

1. Beta-Glucan Content: Oats are rich in beta-glucans, a type of soluble fibre known for its immunomodulatory effects. Beta-glucans help regulate immune responses, potentially reducing chronic inflammation in the body.

2. Antioxidant Compounds: Oats contain various polyphenolic compounds, such as ferulic acid and caffeic acid, which have antioxidant properties. Antioxidants help neutralize free radicals and oxidative stress, which are implicated in inflammation and chronic diseases.

3. Regulation of Gut Health: Oats are a good source of dietary fibre, including soluble fibre, which can promote a healthy gut microbiome. A balanced gut microbiome is crucial for immune function and reducing inflammation throughout the body.

4. Effects on Inflammatory Markers: Research suggests that regular consumption of oats may lower levels of certain inflammatory markers in the body, such as C-reactive protein (CRP) and interleukin-6 (IL-6). These markers are associated with systemic inflammation and various chronic conditions.

Oats offer potential anti-inflammatory benefits primarily through their beta-glucan content, antioxidant compounds, and fibre-rich composition. While not suitable for strict ketogenic diets due to their carb content, oats can still be part of a balanced diet that aims to reduce inflammation and promote overall health. As always, individual tolerance and dietary goals should guide decisions about including oats in your daily eating plan.

The debate between white rice and brown rice often centres around their nutritional value and impact on digestion. Contrary to popular belief, white rice can sometimes be a better choice for those seeking easier digestion and gastrointestinal comfort. This chapter explores the reasons why white rice may be preferable over brown rice in certain digestive contexts.

1. Lower Fibre Content: White rice has had the outer bran and germ layers removed during processing, which reduces its fibre content compared to brown rice. Fibre, while essential for overall health, can be challenging for some individuals to digest, leading to bloating, gas, and discomfort. Gentler on Sensitive Stomachs: For individuals with sensitive digestive systems or conditions such as irritable bowel syndrome (IBS) or Crohn's disease, lower fiber intake from white rice may help reduce symptoms and improve digestive comfort.

2. Reduced Antinutrients: Brown rice contains higher levels of phytic acid, an antinutrient that can bind to minerals like iron, zinc, and calcium, inhibiting their absorption. While phytic acid is present in both types of rice, the processing of white rice reduces its levels, potentially enhancing mineral absorption and overall nutrient bioavailability.

3. Gentler on the Gut: The outer layers of brown rice can contain compounds that may irritate the digestive tract in some individuals. White rice, with its polished grains, lacks these potentially irritating components, making it easier to digest and less likely to cause gastrointestinal distress.

4. Versatility in Digestive Health Conditions: White rice is often recommended as part of a low-residue diet, which limits foods

that are high in fibre and difficult to digest. This diet is commonly prescribed during periods of gastrointestinal inflammation, recovery from surgery, or flare-ups of conditions like diverticulitis or ulcerative colitis.

Choosing between white rice and brown rice for digestion depends largely on individual tolerance and specific health conditions. While brown rice offers higher fibre content and more nutrients, white rice's lower fibre and reduced antinutrients can make it easier on the digestive system for some people. Understanding your body's response to different types of rice and considering your digestive health goals can help you make an informed choice that supports optimal digestion and overall well-being. Always consult with a healthcare professional or registered dietitian for personalized dietary advice tailored to your individual needs and health conditions.

Both dairy and nut milks offer unique benefits that can support gut health and contribute to overall well-being. Understanding their differences and respective advantages can help you choose the best option based on your dietary preferences and health goals. This chapter explores the benefits of both dairy and nut milks in healing the gut.

1.Dairy Milk: Certain dairy products like yogurt and kefir contain probiotics—beneficial bacteria that promote gut health by supporting digestion and immune function. These probiotics can help maintain a healthy balance of gut flora.

Dairy milk is a significant source of calcium and vitamin D, essential nutrients that contribute to bone health and overall immune function. Adequate calcium intake also supports gut health by promoting the integrity of the intestinal lining.

For individuals who are not lactose intolerant or sensitive to dairy proteins (like casein), dairy milk can be easily digested and provide a readily available source of protein and nutrients.

Fermented dairy products such as yogurt and kefir contain beneficial bacteria that aid in digestion and may help alleviate symptoms of digestive disorders like irritable bowel syndrome (IBS) and inflammatory bowel disease (IBD).

2. Nut Milks: like almond milk, coconut milk, and cashew milk are naturally lactose-free, making them suitable alternatives for individuals who are lactose intolerant or sensitive to dairy products.

Nut milks are typically higher in healthy fats, such as monounsaturated and polyunsaturated fats, which can support gut health by reducing inflammation and promoting a healthy microbiome.

Depending on the nut used, nut milks can provide various nutrients such as vitamin E, magnesium, and antioxidants, which have anti-inflammatory properties and support overall immune function.

Nut milks are generally easier to digest compared to dairy milk for many people, particularly those with digestive issues or sensitivities to dairy proteins.

Both dairy and nut milks offer valuable benefits in supporting gut health and overall well-being. Dairy milk provides probiotics, calcium, and vitamin D, which support digestive and immune functions. Nut milks, on the other hand, are lactose-free, rich in healthy fats, and packed with nutrients that can contribute to a balanced diet and improved gut health. Whether you choose dairy or nut milks, selecting options that align with your dietary preferences and digestive needs can help optimize gut health and enhance your overall quality of life.

Filtered water plays a crucial role in maintaining optimal health and enhancing the quality of your meals. This chapter explores why using filtered water is essential for drinking and cooking, highlighting its benefits and practical considerations.

1. Removal of Contaminants: Filters effectively remove impurities such as chlorine, lead, mercury, pesticides, and microbial contaminants from tap water. Eliminating these substances reduces the risk of exposure to harmful toxins and pathogens, supporting overall health.

2. Improving Taste and Odour: Filtered water often tastes and smells better than untreated tap water, enhancing the sensory experience of drinking and cooking. Using clean, pure water can improve the taste and quality of ingredients in recipes, especially in beverages and delicate dishes.

3. Reducing Chemical Exposure: Filters remove chlorine and its by-products, which can irritate the digestive system and disrupt gut microbiota balance. Filtration systems reduce exposure to heavy metals like lead and mercury, which are harmful to the nervous system and overall health.

4. Supporting Digestive Health: Cleaner water helps maintain a healthy gut microbiome by reducing exposure to contaminants that can disrupt microbial balance. Proper hydration with filtered water supports digestion, nutrient absorption, and overall gastrointestinal function.

5. Preserving Nutrients: Using filtered water in cooking preserves the natural flavours and nutrients of ingredients, enhancing the nutritional value of meals. Clean water ensures that contaminants do not leach into food during boiling or steaming processes.

Using filtered water for drinking and cooking is a simple yet impactful step toward improving overall health and culinary quality. By removing contaminants, enhancing taste, supporting digestive health, and promoting environmental sustainability, filtered water contributes to a healthier lifestyle and enjoyable dining experiences. Embrace the benefits of clean, pure water in your daily routines to nourish your body, protect your health, and elevate your culinary creations.

Ceremonial cocoa, often referred to as ceremonial cacao, has gained popularity not only for its rich history rooted in ancient Mesoamerican cultures but also for its potential health benefits and spiritual significance in ceremonial practices. This chapter explores the various benefits of ceremonial cocoa, ranging from its nutritional content to its role in emotional and spiritual well-being.

1. Antioxidant Power: Ceremonial cocoa is packed with antioxidants, specifically flavonoids like epicatechin, catechin, and procyanidins. These compounds help combat oxidative stress, reduce inflammation, and support overall cellular health.

2. Mineral Content: It's rich in essential minerals such as magnesium, iron, zinc, and potassium, which are crucial for various bodily functions including energy production, immune support, and muscle function.

3. Theobromine: Unlike caffeine, which is found in coffee, cocoa contains theobromine—a milder stimulant that provides a gentle energy boost without the jittery effects often associated with caffeine.

4. Health Benefits: Beyond its ceremonial use, incorporating ceremonial cocoa into daily life as a warm beverage or ingredient in recipes can provide ongoing health benefits, promoting cardiovascular health, brain function, and overall well-being.

Ceremonial cocoa offers a multifaceted approach to health and wellness, blending its nutritional richness with emotional, spiritual, and ceremonial significance. Whether enjoyed in a traditional ceremonial context or integrated into modern wellness practices, ceremonial cocoa can enhance mindfulness, promote emotional balance, and support overall health.

Embracing the ancient wisdom and holistic benefits of ceremonial cocoa invites individuals to connect with themselves, their communities, and the natural world in profound and transformative ways.

Ceremonial cocoa, known for its rich cultural history and therapeutic properties, can be a delightful addition to a keto diet. This chapter explores how to incorporate ceremonial cocoa into your ketogenic lifestyle while reaping its nutritional benefits and enjoying its ceremonial and spiritual aspects.

1. Traditional Ceremonial Drink: Prepare ceremonial cocoa traditionally by mixing it with hot water or a dairy-free milk alternative like almond milk or coconut milk. Use a keto-friendly sweetener such as stevia or erythritol if desired, but note that ceremonial cocoa is often enjoyed without sweeteners to fully appreciate its natural flavours.

2. Keto Hot Chocolate: Create a keto-friendly hot chocolate by blending ceremonial cocoa with unsweetened almond milk, a dash of heavy cream or coconut cream, and a keto sweetener. Add a pinch of cinnamon or nutmeg for extra flavour.

3. Cocoa Fat Bombs: Make cocoa-infused fat bombs using ceremonial cocoa powder, coconut oil or butter, and a sweetener like monk fruit or stevia. These treats provide a satisfying dose of healthy fats and can be a convenient snack or dessert on keto.

4. Smoothies and Shakes: Incorporate ceremonial cocoa into keto-friendly smoothies or shakes. Blend it with avocado, spinach, unsweetened almond milk, and a keto protein powder for a nutrient-dense, chocolaty treat.

Incorporating ceremonial cocoa into your keto diet not only adds a deliciously chocolaty element but also enhances your overall wellness through its nutritional richness and ceremonial significance. Whether enjoyed as a traditional drink, keto-friendly hot chocolate, or integrated into smoothies and desserts, ceremonial cocoa offers a versatile and enjoyable way to enrich your ketogenic lifestyle. Embrace its ancient wisdom and modern applications to nourish your body, mind, and spirit while staying true to your keto goals.

Integrating natural sweeteners such as maple syrup and blue agave into a ketogenic diet requires careful consideration due to their carbohydrate content. This chapter explores how you can use these sweeteners sparingly while maintaining ketosis, along with alternatives that fit within the keto framework

1. Maple Syrup: Derived from the sap of maple trees, maple syrup is known for its distinct flavour and natural sweetness. It contains sugars like sucrose, glucose, and fructose, which contribute to its carbohydrate content.

2. Blue Agave: A sweetener extracted from the blue agave plant, primarily grown in Mexico, blue agave syrup is sweeter than maple syrup and is often used as an alternative to refined sugars. It consists mainly of fructose and glucose.

3. Stevia: A natural sweetener derived from the stevia plant, stevia is intensely sweet and has zero calories and zero carbohydrates, making it an excellent choice for those following a ketogenic diet.

4. Erythritol: A sugar alcohol that tastes similar to sugar but has minimal impact on blood sugar and insulin levels. Erythritol is often used in baking and cooking as a keto-friendly sweetener.

5. Monk Fruit Extract: Made from the monk fruit, this sweetener is also zero-calorie and does not raise blood sugar levels. It's available in liquid or powder form and can be used as a substitute for sugar in various keto recipes.

Incorporating natural sweeteners like maple syrup and blue agave into a ketogenic diet requires moderation and awareness of their carbohydrate content. While these sweeteners can add flavour and variety to keto-friendly recipes, it's essential to balance their use with other keto-approved sweeteners that have minimal impact on blood sugar levels. By understanding portion control, exploring keto-friendly alternatives, and practicing mindful consumption, you can enjoy occasional sweetness while staying on track with your ketogenic goals and maintaining a healthy lifestyle.

Living with silent reflux had been a constant challenge in my life for almost a year, silently eroding my enjoyment of meals and disrupting my sleep with persistent discomfort. Despite trying various medications and dietary adjustments, the burning sensation in my throat and the nagging feeling of indigestion persisted, casting a shadow over my daily routines.

One day, exhausted from sleepless nights and frustrated with recurring symptoms, I stumbled upon a conversation about Deglycyrrhizinated Licorice (DGL). Intrigued by the possibility of a natural remedy, I delved into research to understand how DGL could potentially offer relief from silent reflux, also known as laryngopharyngeal reflux (LPR).

DGL, unlike regular licorice, has undergone a process to remove glycyrrhizin, which can elevate blood pressure and cause potassium loss. This made DGL a safer option for long-term use to support digestive health and soothe the mucous membranes of the throat and oesophagus.

I decided to give DGL a try, starting with chewable tablets that I would take before meals. The gentle coating of DGL on my throat and stomach lining provided immediate relief from the burning sensation and discomfort that had plagued me for so long. It was as if a soothing balm had been applied to my irritated digestive tract, allowing me to eat without fear of triggering reflux symptoms.

As I continued to incorporate DGL into my daily routine, I noticed significant improvements in my silent reflux symptoms. The frequency and severity of flare-ups diminished, and I regained the ability to enjoy meals without the looming dread of discomfort afterward. Even my sleep improved, as the quiet nights free from reflux-induced coughing and throat irritation became more frequent.

Inspired by my own experience with DGL, I began sharing my journey with friends and family who also struggled with digestive issues. Many were surprised to learn about the effectiveness of DGL in managing silent reflux, and some decided to try it themselves with positive results.

Today, DGL has become an essential part of my wellness regimen, offering me a natural and effective way to manage silent reflux and support my digestive health. I no longer feel held back by the symptoms that once dominated my life, and I am grateful for the relief and freedom that DGL has provided.

My journey with DGL is a testament to the power of natural remedies in achieving and maintaining digestive wellness. It has taught me the importance of listening to my body and seeking gentle yet effective solutions that support long-term health and well-being.

During my research, I learned about Colostrum and the potential healing benefits for the gut. Colostrum is not only essential for nourishing newborns but also holds incredible healing properties for adults, particularly for gut health. Colostrum is rich in bioactive compounds such as immunoglobulins, growth factors, and cytokines. These components play a crucial role in supporting the health and integrity of the gastrointestinal tract.

1. Supports Gut Barrier Function: Colostrum contains immunoglobulins and lactoferrin, which help maintain the integrity of the gut barrier. This barrier is crucial in preventing harmful substances from crossing into the bloodstream and triggering immune responses.

2. Promotes Gut Microbiota Balance: The growth factors in colostrum support the growth of beneficial bacteria in the gut, such as Bifidobacteria and Lactobacilli. A balanced gut microbiota is essential for digestive health and overall well-being.

3. Enhances Immune Function in the Gut: Immunoglobulins and other immune factors in colostrum help to strengthen the immune defences within the gut. This can reduce susceptibility to infections and inflammatory conditions that affect the digestive system.

4. Supports Healing of Gut Lining: Colostrum contains factors that promote tissue repair and regeneration. This can be beneficial for individuals with conditions such as leaky gut syndrome or gastrointestinal inflammation, helping to restore and heal the mucosal lining of the intestines.

5. Anti-Inflammatory Properties: Components like lactoferrin and cytokines in colostrum have anti-inflammatory effects, which can help alleviate inflammation in the gut and reduce symptoms associated with inflammatory bowel diseases (IBD) like Crohn's

disease and ulcerative colitis.

As I started taking colostrum regularly, I began to notice gradual improvements in my digestive health. The bloating that had once plagued me diminished, and my bowel movements became more regular and comfortable. Over time, I felt a renewed sense of vitality and well-being, grateful for the transformative effects of colostrum on my gut health.

Whilst suffering a particularly nasty bout of silent reflux, I found myself on a journey of discovery—an exploration that would ultimately lead me to embrace the transformative power of L-glutamine for my gut health.

For years, I had struggled silently with digestive discomfort. Bloating, irregularity, and occasional bouts of discomfort after meals had become a constant companion, casting a shadow over my daily life. Despite countless visits to doctors and attempts at dietary adjustments, relief seemed elusive.

One day, amidst my quest for answers, I stumbled upon information about L-glutamine—a humble amino acid known for its profound role in supporting gastrointestinal health. Intrigued by its potential benefits, I delved deeper into research, eager to understand how L-glutamine could offer solace to my troubled digestive system.

L-glutamine, I learned, is not merely a building block of protein but a crucial nutrient for maintaining the integrity of the intestinal lining. It serves as fuel for the cells that line the digestive tract, supporting their growth, repair, and function. This is particularly vital in conditions where the gut lining may be compromised, such as leaky gut syndrome or inflammatory bowel diseases.

Armed with newfound knowledge and hope, I decided to incorporate L-glutamine supplements into my daily routine. I opted for a high-quality source, ensuring purity and potency to maximize its therapeutic benefits.

As I began taking L-glutamine regularly, I started to notice subtle yet significant changes in my digestive health. The uncomfortable bloating that had once plagued me gradually subsided. My bowel movements became more regular and comfortable, signalling a newfound balance within my gut ecosystem.

The real turning point came when I noticed a reduction in inflammation and irritation. The nagging discomfort after meals diminished, replaced by a soothing sensation that hinted at healing from within. I felt more energized and less weighed down by digestive woes, reclaiming a sense of vitality that had eluded me for so long.

Inspired by my progress, I began to complement L-glutamine supplementation with mindful eating practices and a balanced diet rich in whole foods. I prioritized gut-friendly nutrients and avoided triggers that could exacerbate digestive symptoms. With each wholesome meal, I nurtured my gut health and honoured the intricate connection between nutrition and well-being.

As word of my journey spread within my community, I found myself surrounded by others who sought solace from similar digestive challenges. I shared my experiences with L-glutamine, offering guidance and support to those embarking on their own paths to gut healing. Together, we celebrated small victories and embraced the promise of a healthier tomorrow.

Today, L-glutamine remains an integral part of my wellness regimen—a steadfast ally in my ongoing quest for digestive harmony. It has taught me the profound impact of nurturing my gut health from within, fostering resilience and vitality that extend far beyond physical comfort.

My journey with L-glutamine is a testament to the power of natural remedies in restoring balance and reclaiming wellness. It has reaffirmed my belief in the body's innate capacity to heal when provided with the right support and nourishment.

In our pursuit of health and wellness, it's crucial to emphasize the importance of balance and moderation. While adopting healthy eating habits is beneficial, rigid rules and strict diets can sometimes overshadow the joy and satisfaction that food brings to our lives. This chapter explores the significance of maintaining a mindful balance, enjoying everything in moderation, and embracing life fully.

1. Variety and Nutrient Density: Consuming a diverse range of foods ensures that we obtain a wide spectrum of nutrients essential for overall health and well-being. Aim to include a variety of fruits, vegetables, whole grains, lean proteins, and healthy fats in your daily meals. This approach not only promotes nutritional balance but also adds excitement and enjoyment to eating.

2. Flexibility and Adaptability: Adopt a flexible mindset towards dietary choices, allowing room for occasional indulgences without guilt or stress. Incorporate foods you love in moderation, understanding that occasional treats can be part of a balanced diet. Listen to your body's cues of hunger and fullness to guide your eating habits.

3. Portion Control and Awareness: Practice mindful eating by paying attention to portion sizes and savouring each bite. Use smaller plates, take your time to chew thoroughly, and pause between bites to assess hunger levels. This mindful approach can prevent overeating and promote better digestion.

4. Enjoyment and Pleasure: Allow yourself to enjoy foods you love without guilt, focusing on the pleasure and satisfaction they bring. Plan occasional treats or special meals, savouring the experience and being fully present in the moment. This balanced approach fosters a positive relationship with food and supports

emotional well-being.

Achieving a balanced approach to eating involves mindfulness, moderation, and a holistic perspective on health and happiness. By embracing variety in your diet, practicing moderation with indulgences, and fully enjoying life's experiences, you can cultivate a sustainable and enriching lifestyle. Remember, every person's journey to wellness is unique, and finding your own balance requires listening to your body and honouring your individual needs and preferences. Strive for a harmonious relationship with food and life, where nourishment, enjoyment, and well-being coexist in harmony.

Maintaining weight loss isn't just about short-term diets but rather finding a sustainable eating lifestyle that suits your body's needs and preferences. This chapter explores the importance of tweaking your eating habits to support weight maintenance effectively.

1. Personalized Approach: Recognize that each person's metabolism, nutritional requirements, and response to different foods are unique. Pay attention to how your body responds to certain foods, portion sizes, and eating patterns to identify what works best for you.

2. Nutrient Density: Aim for a diet rich in nutrient-dense foods, including lean proteins, whole grains, fruits, vegetables, healthy fats, and adequate hydration. Choose foods that provide satiety and satisfaction to prevent overeating and maintain energy levels throughout the day.

3. Meal Frequency and Timing: Eat regular meals and snacks throughout the day to maintain stable blood sugar levels and prevent extreme hunger. Consider your daily schedule and preferences when planning meals to ensure consistency and prevent erratic eating patterns.

Maintaining weight loss and achieving long-term health require a personalized approach to eating that aligns with your body's needs, preferences, and lifestyle. By adopting a balanced and flexible eating plan, focusing on nutrient density, practicing portion control, and enjoying food in moderation, you can establish sustainable habits that support your weight maintenance goals effectively. Remember, the journey to optimal health is a continuous process of self-discovery and adjustment, where listening to your body and prioritizing consistency are key to long-term success

Maintaining a food journal can be a powerful tool for identifying trigger foods, understanding eating habits, and promoting mindful eating practices. This chapter explores the benefits of keeping a food journal specifically for identifying trigger foods and provides practical strategies for effective journaling.

1. Awareness and Accountability: Recording everything you eat and drink increases awareness of your dietary habits and patterns. Journalling also helps pinpoint specific foods or situations that trigger cravings, emotional eating, or overeating episodes.

2. Behavioural Insights: Detect patterns in eating behaviours, such as times of day, emotional states, or environmental cues associated with consuming trigger foods and recognize emotional triggers and associations with certain foods, such as stress eating or reward-based eating habits.

Keeping a food journal is a valuable tool for identifying trigger foods, understanding eating behaviours, and promoting mindful choices. By documenting meals, snacks, emotions, and physical responses, you can gain insights into your dietary habits and their impact on overall well-being. Utilize the data collected to make informed decisions, set achievable goals, and cultivate a balanced approach to eating that supports long-term health and wellness. Remember, the process of self-discovery through food journaling is a journey towards fostering a healthier relationship with food and achieving personal dietary goals.

Meal prepping is not just a convenient habit; it can significantly contribute to healing your gut and resetting your overall health. This chapter explores why meal prepping is imperative for gut health, how it supports a health reset, and practical tips for effective meal preparation. If I didn't plan ahead and take lunch to work every day. I would soon enough reach for unhealthy alternatives that would trigger my symptoms.

1. Nutrient-Dense Choices: Meal prepping encourages the use of whole, unprocessed ingredients rich in fibre, vitamins, and minerals essential for gut health. Plan meals that incorporate a variety of vegetables, fruits, lean proteins, healthy fats, and whole grains to support digestive function and microbial diversity.

2. Consistency and Routine: Establishing a meal prepping routine promotes consistent eating times and balanced meals, which can aid digestion and nutrient absorption. By preparing meals in advance, you reduce the temptation to opt for convenience foods that may be detrimental to gut health.

3. Controlled Ingredients: Prepare meals with minimal additives, preservatives, and artificial ingredients that can disrupt gut microbiota and contribute to inflammation. Select ingredients known for their gut-supporting properties, such as probiotic-rich foods (like yogurt and fermented vegetables) and prebiotic foods (like oats, bananas, and garlic).

4. Portion Control and Balanced Meals: Portion meals appropriately to prevent overeating and support digestive comfort. Ensure meals contain a balance of carbohydrates, proteins, and fats to sustain energy levels and support overall health.

Meal prepping is a proactive approach to supporting gut

health and achieving a health reset by promoting nutrient-dense, balanced meals. By incorporating whole foods, controlling ingredients, and establishing a routine, you can enhance digestive function, reduce inflammation, and support overall well-being. Embrace meal prepping as a tool for self-care and empowerment on your journey toward improved gut health and long-term vitality.

Once upon a time, there was a person who struggled with persistent health challenges – that person was me. Despite trying various treatments and lifestyle changes, I found myself grappling with ongoing issues that impacted my daily life. Among these struggles was a persistent problem with digestion and discomfort in the abdominal area.

After extensive research and consultation with healthcare professionals, stumbled upon information about the potential benefits of enemas for digestive health. Intrigued by the possibility of finding relief, I cautiously approached the idea and decided to give it a try under medical supervision.

At first, the process seemed daunting and unfamiliar. I meticulously followed the instructions provided by my healthcare provider, ensuring every step was carried out with precision and care. Gradually, I began to notice subtle improvements in my digestion. The discomfort that had become a constant companion started to ease, and I felt lighter and more comfortable after each session.

Encouraged by these initial positive outcomes, I integrated regular enemas into my wellness routine. Over time, the benefits became more pronounced. I experienced fewer episodes of bloating and indigestion, and my overall energy levels improved. This newfound relief spurred me on to continue with my regimen diligently.

As I persisted with the treatment, I also made complementary adjustments to my diet and lifestyle. I focused on consuming more fibre-rich foods, staying hydrated, and incorporating gentle exercise into my daily routine. These holistic efforts worked synergistically with the enemas, contributing to sustained improvements in my digestive health and overall well-being.

With each passing month, I felt more empowered and in control of my health journey. The discomfort that once overshadowed my days gradually became a distant memory. I shared my experiences cautiously with friends and family, emphasizing the importance of informed decision-making and personalized healthcare approaches.

While my journey wasn't without challenges or setbacks, I remained committed to maintaining a balanced approach to my health. I continued to consult with healthcare professionals regularly, ensuring I was on the right track and adjusting my regimen as necessary.

In the end, my story wasn't just about finding relief through enemas, but about the journey of self-discovery and perseverance in pursuit of better health. It underscored the importance of listening to one's body, seeking informed medical advice, and taking proactive steps towards holistic well-being

Enemas and colonic irrigation are practices that involve flushing liquid into the rectum for cleansing purposes. While they are sometimes promoted for digestive health, their benefits and risks should be carefully considered:

1. Constipation Relief: Enemas can provide immediate relief from constipation by softening stool and promoting bowel movements. However, frequent use may lead to dependence and disrupt natural bowel function.

2. Detoxification Claims: Advocates suggest that colonic irrigation removes toxins from the colon, but there's limited scientific evidence to support this. The colon naturally eliminates waste products, and the liver and kidneys primarily handle detoxification.

3. Hydration and Electrolyte Balance: Enemas and colonic irrigation can affect fluid and electrolyte balance in the body. Proper hydration and electrolyte levels are crucial for overall health, and excessive use can lead to imbalance.

In conclusion, while enemas and colonic irrigation may offer short-term relief for constipation, claims about detoxification and long-term digestive health benefits are not well-supported by scientific evidence. It's essential to weigh the potential risks and benefits carefully and seek medical advice before starting any regimen involving these practices.

In the labyrinth of dietary trends and wellness advice, I found myself navigating a sea of options in search of relief from persistent health challenges. Despite numerous attempts with various diets and protocols, my symptoms persisted—a cycle of discomfort, fatigue, and frustration. It wasn't until I discovered the carnivore reset that I embarked on a transformative journey towards healing.

The concept of a carnivore reset intrigued me—a dietary approach centred around animal-based foods, primarily meat, fish, and animal fats, while eliminating plant-based foods and carbohydrates. At first glance, it seemed counterintuitive, challenging conventional wisdom about balanced diets rich in fruits, vegetables, and whole grains. Yet, driven by desperation and curiosity, I decided to embark on this unconventional path.

As I embarked on the carnivore reset, I embraced a new way of eating that prioritised nutrient-dense animal foods. My meals consisted of high-quality cuts of beef, lamb, poultry, and fatty fish, prepared simply and seasoned minimally. Gone were the grains, legumes, fruits, and vegetables that once dominated my plate—a radical departure from my previous dietary habits.

In the initial days, my body underwent a period of adjustment, adapting to the absence of familiar foods and the influx of animal-based nutrients. Surprisingly, I began to notice subtle improvements. The persistent bloating and digestive discomfort that plagued me for years started to diminish. My energy levels stabilized, and mental clarity replaced the brain fog that had clouded my thoughts.

Intrigued by these early signs of progress, I continued to explore the carnivore reset with dedication and mindfulness. I learned that animal-based foods provide essential nutrients such as high-quality protein, B vitamins, iron, and zinc—all crucial for optimal health and vitality. The absence of potentially irritating plant compounds allowed my gut to rest and heal, reducing inflammation and supporting digestive function.

As weeks turned into months on the carnivore reset, I experienced profound transformations in my health and well-being. The nagging symptoms that once overshadowed my daily life became distant memories. I regained a sense of control over my health, feeling empowered by the simplicity and efficacy of this dietary approach.

Beyond physical improvements, I discovered unexpected benefits of mental resilience and emotional stability. Freed from the rollercoaster of sugar highs and crashes, I found myself more grounded and focused—a testament to the profound impact of diet on overall wellness.

Reflecting on my journey with the carnivore reset, I realised the power of listening to my body's unique needs and challenging conventional norms. By embracing a diet rich in animal-based nutrients and eliminating potential triggers, I not only embarked on a path to healing but also rediscovered a renewed sense of vitality and well-being. My journey with the carnivore reset continues to inspire me to prioritize holistic health practices and embrace the transformative potential of dietary choices in achieving optimal wellness.

Starting with a carnivore reset for 4 weeks and then transitioning into a keto diet or anti-inflammatory can be a structured approach to resetting your metabolism and transitioning into a sustainable healthy gut eating plan. Here's a guide to help you get started:

Week 1:

1. Plan Your Meals: Focus on animal-based foods such as meat, fish, eggs, and dairy (if tolerated). Avoid all plant-based foods including vegetables, fruits, grains, legumes, and nuts.

2. Stay Hydrated: Drink plenty of water throughout the day to stay hydrated and support digestion.

3. Monitor Your Body: Pay attention to how your body responds to the diet change. Note any changes in energy levels, digestion, or overall well-being.

Week 2:

1. Variety in Meat: Include a variety of meats such as beef, chicken, pork, lamb, and fish to ensure you're getting a range of nutrients.

2. Adjust Fat Intake: Experiment with different fat sources like fatty cuts of meat, butter, and tallow to find what works best for you.

3. Supplements: Consider adding electrolytes or magnesium if needed, as a purely carnivorous diet can sometimes require additional supplementation.

Week 3:

1. Meal Timing: Experiment with meal timing that suits your lifestyle, whether it's two larger meals or multiple smaller ones throughout the day.

2.*Monitor Health Indicator: Keep an eye on cholesterol levels, blood pressure, and other health indicators if you have preexisting conditions.

3. Consultation: If you have any concerns about your diet or health, consult with a healthcare professional.

Week 4:

1. Evaluate Your Progress: Assess how you feel physically and mentally after completing four weeks on a carnivore diet.

2. Transition Plan: Begin planning your transition to a keto diet by gradually reintroducing low-carb vegetables and healthy fats.

Week 5 and Beyond:

1. Reintroduce Vegetables and grains: Start incorporating low-carb vegetables such as leafy greens, broccoli, cauliflower, and zucchini back into your diet. Slowly add white rice, oats, chia and quinoa if you are choosing to utilise the anti-inflammatory diet.

2. Healthy Fats: Include healthy fats like avocado, olive oil, nuts (if tolerated), and seeds to increase your fat intake while keeping carbohydrates low.

3. Keep Track: Monitor your macronutrient intake to ensure you're staying within the keto range of 70-75% fat, 20-25% protein, and 5-10% carbohydrates if you have chosen keto rather than anti-inflammatory.

4. Meal Planning: Plan your meals to maintain a balance of protein, fats, and low-carb vegetables. Use keto-friendly recipes for variety and to ensure you're getting adequate nutrients.

5. Long-Term Sustainability: Focus on creating a sustainable eating pattern that works for your lifestyle and supports your health goals.

6. Stay Hydrated: Continue to drink plenty of water to support digestion and overall well-being.

By following this structured approach of starting with a carnivore reset and then transitioning to a keto or anti-inflammatory diet, you can effectively reset your metabolism, improve nutrient absorption, and achieve your health and wellness goals. Remember, individual responses to dietary changes vary, so always listen to your body and consult with a healthcare professional if you have any concerns.

Carnivore - Creating a one-week meal plan focused on red meat and broth in a carnivore style diet involves simplicity and strategic planning. Here's a sample meal plan that emphasizes nutrient-dense red meat and nourishing bone broth:

Week 1:

Day 1:

- **Breakfast:** Scrambled eggs cooked in beef tallow

- **Lunch:** Ribeye steak with a side of bone broth

- **Dinner:** Lamb chops with melted butter

Day 2:

- **Breakfast:** Bacon and eggs

- **Lunch:** Ground beef patties cooked in lard

- **Dinner:** Beef short ribs with bone marrow

Day 3:

- **Breakfast:** Sausages (without fillers) and scrambled eggs

- **Lunch:** Beef liver (if desired) cooked in beef tallow

- **Dinner:** Grilled pork chops with bone broth

Day 4:

- **Breakfast:** Omelette with cheese (if tolerated)

- **Lunch:** Braised beef shank with bone broth

- **Dinner:** Venison steak with herb butter

Day 5:

- **Breakfast:** Bacon and fried eggs

- **Lunch:** Bison burger patties cooked in lard

- **Dinner:** Beef brisket with au jus

Day 6:

- **Breakfast:** Sausage links and scrambled eggs

- **Lunch:** Beef tongue (if desired) with bone broth

- **Dinner:** Lamb shoulder chops with melted ghee

Day 7:

- **Breakfast:** Pork belly slices and eggs

- **Lunch:** Beef chuck roast with bone broth

- **Dinner:** Prime rib roast with pan drippings

Week 2:

Day 8:

- **Breakfast:** Scrambled eggs cooked in butter

- **Lunch:** Grilled chicken thighs

- **Dinner:** Beef bone broth with beef liver and a side of full-fat yogurt

Day 9:

- **Breakfast:** Bacon and fried eggs

- **Lunch:** Pork chops cooked in lard

- **Dinner:** Lamb stew with bone broth and a serving of fermented cottage cheese

Day 10:

- **Breakfast:** Omelette with cheese (if tolerated)

- **Lunch:** Roast turkey breast cooked in butter

- **Dinner:** Beef chuck roast with beef bone broth and a side of kefir

Day 11:

- **Breakfast:** Sausage links and scrambled eggs

- **Lunch:** Grilled salmon fillet

- **Dinner:** Beef liver (if desired) cooked in beef tallow and a serving of fermented yogurt

Day 12:

- **Breakfast:** Fried eggs and bacon

- **Lunch:** Chicken drumsticks cooked in duck fat

- **Dinner:** Beef brisket with beef bone broth and a side of fermented cream cheese

Day 13:

- **Breakfast:** Omelette with ham (if desired) and cheese (if tolerated)

- **Lunch:** Grilled shrimp with melted butter

- **Dinner:** Prime ribeye steak with au jus and a serving of fermented sour cream

Day 14:

- **Breakfast:** Sausage patties and fried eggs

- **Lunch:** Roast duck breast

- **Dinner:** Beef bone broth with beef meatballs and a side of fermented goat cheese

KETO - Creating a two-week keto meal plan that emphasizes whole foods, includes fermented foods, avoids inflammatory and processed foods can be both nutritious and delicious. Here's a balanced plan:

Week 1:

Day 1:

- **Breakfast:** Scrambled eggs with spinach cooked in olive oil

- **Lunch:** Grilled chicken breast with a side salad (lettuce, cucumber, tomatoes) and olive oil dressing

- **Dinner:** Baked salmon with steamed broccoli and a dollop of sauerkraut

Day 2:

- **Breakfast:** Greek yogurt with mixed berries (blueberries, strawberries) and a sprinkle of chia seeds

- **Lunch:** Beef stir-fry (beef strips, bell peppers, onions) cooked in coconut oil

- **Dinner:** Zucchini noodles (zoodles) with creamy Alfredo sauce (made with heavy cream and Parmesan cheese)

Day 3:

- **Breakfast:** Chia seed pudding made with coconut milk, topped with sliced almonds and raspberries

- **Lunch:** Turkey lettuce wraps with avocado, cucumber, and a side of kimchi

- **Dinner:** Baked chicken thighs with roasted asparagus and a side of fermented pickles

Day 4:

- **Breakfast:** Smoothie with spinach, avocado, coconut milk, and protein powder (keto-friendly)

- **Lunch:** Cauliflower rice with shrimp, broccoli, and a drizzle of tamari sauce (gluten-free soy sauce)

- **Dinner:** Pork tenderloin with roasted Brussels sprouts and a small serving of sauerkraut

Day 5:

- **Breakfast:** Omelette with cheese, mushrooms, and spinach cooked in butter

- **Lunch:** Tuna salad (canned tuna, mayo, celery, and pickles) in lettuce wraps

- **Dinner:** Grilled steak with a side of steamed green beans and fermented carrots

Day 6:

- **Breakfast:** Coconut flour pancakes topped with whipped cream and a few strawberries

- **Lunch:** Egg salad (hard-boiled eggs, mayo, mustard) on a bed of arugula

- **Dinner:** Baked cod with lemon butter sauce, served with sautéed spinach and a side of fermented beetroot

Day 7:

- **Breakfast:** Avocado stuffed with scrambled eggs and salsa

- **Lunch:** Chicken Caesar salad (grilled chicken, romaine lettuce, Parmesan cheese, Caesar dressing)

- **Dinner:** Beef kabobs with bell peppers and onions, served with a side of fermented cabbage

Week 2:

Day 8:

- **Breakfast:** Smoothie bowl with avocado, spinach, coconut milk, and topped with hemp seeds and almonds
- **Lunch:** Turkey and avocado lettuce wraps with a side of fermented vegetables
- **Dinner:** Baked salmon with cauliflower mash and a dollop of sauerkraut

Day 9:

- **Breakfast:** Greek yogurt with sliced almonds, flaxseeds, and a handful of raspberries
- **Lunch:** Beef taco bowl (ground beef, lettuce, avocado, salsa, sour cream)
- **Dinner:** Chicken thighs with roasted Brussels sprouts and fermented pickles

Day 10:

- **Breakfast:** Scrambled eggs with spinach cooked in olive oil
- **Lunch:** Cauliflower rice with shrimp, broccoli, and a drizzle of tamari sauce
- **Dinner:** Pork chops with steamed asparagus and a side of fermented carrots

Day 11:

- **Breakfast:** Chia seed pudding with coconut milk, topped with sliced almonds and blueberries

- **Lunch:** Tuna salad in lettuce wraps with a side of kimchi

- **Dinner:** Grilled steak with roasted cauliflower and sauerkraut

Day 12:

- **Breakfast:** Smoothie with spinach, avocado, coconut milk, and protein powder

- **Lunch:** Turkey lettuce wraps with avocado and fermented pickles

- **Dinner:** Baked cod with lemon butter sauce, served with sautéed spinach and fermented beetroot

Day 13:

- **Breakfast:** Coconut flour pancakes with whipped cream and a few strawberries

- **Lunch:** Egg salad on a bed of arugula with fermented vegetables

- **Dinner:** Chicken thighs with roasted broccoli and a side of fermented cabbage

Day 14:

- **Breakfast:** Avocado stuffed with scrambled eggs and salsa

- **Lunch:** Chicken Caesar salad with Parmesan cheese, Caesar dressing, and fermented vegetables

- **Dinner:** Beef kabobs with bell peppers and onions, served with sautéed spinach

This meal plan provides a balanced approach to a keto diet while focusing on whole, nutrient-dense foods and avoiding inflammatory and processed ingredients. Adjust portion sizes and specific foods based on individual preferences and dietary needs.

Anti-inflammatory - Here's a 2-week anti-inflammatory meal plan that incorporates oats while eliminating bread:

Week 1

Day 1:

- **Breakfast:** Overnight oats with almond milk, topped with berries, chia seeds, and a drizzle of honey.
- **Lunch:** Quinoa salad with spinach, cherry tomatoes, cucumber, avocado, and grilled chicken.
- **Dinner:** Baked salmon with quinoa pilaf and steamed broccoli.

Day 2:

- **Breakfast:** Smoothie with spinach, kale, banana, oats, and almond butter.
- **Lunch:** Lentil and vegetable soup with a side of mixed greens.
- **Dinner:** Grilled turkey breast with roasted sweet potatoes and asparagus.

Day 3:

- **Breakfast:** Chia pudding with coconut milk, topped with mango and sliced almonds.
- **Lunch:** Chickpea and kale salad with lemon tahini dressing.
- **Dinner:** Stir-fried tofu with bell peppers, broccoli, and brown rice.

Day 4:

- **Breakfast:** Greek yogurt with oats, nuts, and fresh berries.
- **Lunch:** Quinoa-stuffed bell peppers with a side of mixed greens.
- **Dinner:** Baked chicken thighs with quinoa tabbouleh and roasted Brussels sprouts.

Day 5:

- **Breakfast:** Smoothie bowl with mixed berries, spinach, oats, and a sprinkle of hemp seeds.
- **Lunch:** Mixed greens salad with grilled shrimp, avocado, tomatoes, and a drizzle of olive oil.
- **Dinner:** Grilled salmon with quinoa pilaf and steamed green beans.

Week 2

Day 6:

- **Breakfast:** Overnight oats with almond milk, topped with sliced banana, walnuts, and a drizzle of maple syrup.
- **Lunch:** Lentil and vegetable curry with brown rice.
- **Dinner:** Turkey meatballs with zucchini noodles and marinara sauce.

Day 7:

- **Breakfast:** Smoothie with oats, kale, pineapple, ginger, and

Greek yogurt.

- **Lunch:** Quinoa salad with mixed greens, cucumber, feta cheese, and a lemon vinaigrette.

- **Dinner:** Baked cod with quinoa pilaf and sautéed spinach.

Day 8:

- **Breakfast:** Chia pudding with almond milk, topped with sliced peaches and a sprinkle of cinnamon.

- **Lunch:** Chickpea and kale salad with roasted vegetables and a tahini dressing.

- **Dinner:** Grilled chicken breast with quinoa tabbouleh and steamed asparagus.

Day 9:

- **Breakfast:** Yogurt parfait with oats, Greek yogurt, mixed berries, and a drizzle of honey.

- **Lunch:** Quinoa and black bean burrito bowl with salsa, avocado, and cilantro.

- **Dinner:** Baked salmon with quinoa pilaf and roasted Brussels sprouts.

Day 10:

- **Breakfast:** Smoothie bowl with oats, spinach, mango, almond butter, and coconut flakes.

- **Lunch:** Lentil soup with a side of mixed greens.

- **Dinner:** Grilled shrimp skewers with quinoa and steamed broccoli.

This meal plan emphasizes whole, nutrient-dense foods while eliminating bread and incorporating oats for their fiber and anti-inflammatory benefits. Adjust portion sizes and specific foods based on individual preferences, dietary restrictions, and health goals. Always consult with a healthcare professional or registered dietitian before making significant changes to your diet, especially if you have specific health concerns or conditions.

Carnivore

Protein Sources:

- Ribeye steak

- Beef sirloin

- Ground beef (preferably grass-fed)

- Lamb chops

- Pork chops

- Bacon (uncured, sugar-free)

- Chicken thighs

- Turkey breast

- Salmon fillets

- Shrimp

- Eggs (preferably pasture-raised)

Organ Meats (optional):

- Beef liver

- Chicken liver

- Heart (beef, chicken, etc.)

Dairy (if tolerated):

- Full-fat Greek yogurt (plain, no added sugars)

- Full-fat cottage cheese

- Heavy cream (for coffee or cooking)

Fats:

- Grass-fed butter

- Ghee (clarified butter)

- Lard (preferably from pastured pigs)

- Tallow (beef fat)

- Duck fat

Broth and Stock:
- Beef bone broth (preferably homemade or low-sodium)

- Chicken bone broth (preferably homemade or low-sodium)

Fermented Foods:
- Sauerkraut (check for no added sugars)

- Kimchi

- Pickles (check for no added sugars)

- Fermented dairy products (if tolerated)

Condiments and Seasonings:
- Sea salt (for seasoning)

- Black pepper (for seasoning)

- Dijon mustard (check for no added sugars)

- Tamari sauce (gluten-free soy sauce, in moderation)

- Apple cider vinegar (for dressings)

Beverages:
- Water (sparkling or still)

- Herbal teas (caffeine-free)

Optional Snacks (if desired):

- Beef jerky (no added sugars)

- Pork rinds (plain)

Keto

Protein Sources:

- Salmon

- Sardines

- Mackerel

- Trout

- Grass-fed beef

- Lamb

- Pasture-raised chicken

- Turkey

- Eggs (preferably pasture-raised)

Vegetables (Low-Carb):

- Spinach

- Kale

- Swiss chard

- Arugula

- Broccoli

- Cauliflower

- Brussels sprouts

- Asparagus

- Zucchini

- Bell peppers (green, red, yellow)

Healthy Fats:

- Avocado

- Avocado oil

- Olive oil (extra virgin)

- Coconut oil

- Grass-fed butter

- Ghee (clarified butter)

- MCT oil (medium-chain triglycerides)

Nuts and Seeds (in moderation):
- Almonds

- Walnuts

- Chia seeds

- Flaxseeds

- Hemp seeds

- Macadamia nuts

Berries (Low-Sugar):
- Blueberries

- Raspberries

- Strawberries

Herbs and Spices:
- Turmeric

- Ginger

- Garlic

- Basil

- Cilantro

- Parsley

- Rosemary
- Thyme

Beverages:
- Water (still or sparkling)
- Herbal teas (caffeine-free)
- Green tea (anti-inflammatory properties)

Dairy (if tolerated):
- Full-fat Greek yogurt (plain, no added sugars)
- Cheese (preferably hard cheeses like cheddar, mozzarella, or feta)
- Heavy cream (for coffee or cooking)
- Kefir

Condiments and Extras:
- Apple cider vinegar (raw, unfiltered)
- Sea salt (preferably Himalayan or Celtic sea salt)
- Black pepper
- Lemon (for flavoring)

Supplements (optional):
- Omega-3 fatty acids (fish oil or algae oil)
- Magnesium
- Vitamin D (if deficient)

Miscellaneous:
- Bone broth (homemade or store-bought, low-sodium)
- Olives (green or black)

- Pickles (check for no added sugars)

Anti-inflammatory

Vegetables:
- Spinach

- Kale

- Broccoli

- Cauliflower

- Brussels sprouts

- Bell peppers

- Cucumber

- Avocado

- Sweet potatoes

Fruits:
- Berries (strawberries, blueberries, raspberries)

- Oranges

- Lemons

- Apples

- Mango

- Pineapple

- Peaches

Protein:
- Salmon

- Chicken breasts/thighs

- Turkey breast

- Tofu

- Eggs

Legumes and Grains:

- Oats (rolled or steel-cut)

- Quinoa

- Lentils

- Chickpeas

Nuts and Seeds:

- Almonds

- Walnuts

- Chia seeds

- Flaxseeds

- Pumpkin seeds

Dairy and Alternatives:

- Greek yogurt (unsweetened)

- Sour cream

- Cottage cheese

- Kefir

- Almond milk or coconut milk (unsweetened)

Herbs and Spices:

- Turmeric

- Ginger

- Garlic

- Cinnamon

- Basil

- Parsley

- Cilantro

Oils and Condiments:
- Extra virgin olive oil

- Avocado oil

- Coconut oil

- Tahini

- Balsamic vinegar

Miscellaneous:
- Dark chocolate (70% cocoa or higher)

- Green tea

- Herbal teas (such as chamomile or ginger)

Stacked Carnivore Burgers Recipe

Ingredients:

- pork belly/bacon
- ground beef (or other burger meat)
- cheese
- egg
- pulled pork/shredded beef
- salt
(Note: We love to throw a pork shoulder or chuck roast sprinkled with salt in the crockpot over the weekend and eat on it throughout the week)

Directions:

- Cook salted pork belly or bacon in pan and set aside on plate.
- Pan fry burger in bacon grease and salt both sides at end. [Bonus if you add pureed liver to your burger meat!]
- Place burger on plate and cover with thick slice of cheese while hot.
- Fry an egg in remaining grease and place on top of cheese.
- Lastly, fry up previously cooked pulled pork or shredded beef until browned or slightly crispy, then place on top of burger stack. This process helps to soak up all the fat in the pan.

Salmon With Cream Cheese Sauce

Ingredients:

- Fresh caught salmon
- 4 ounces cream cheese
- 1/2 cup chicken stock
- salt
- pepper (optional)

Directions:

- Cook salmon to your liking.
- Add all ingredients to a small spot and whisk at medium heat until combined and creamy.

Carnivore Flat Bread

Ingredients:

- 3 eggs
- ¾ cup Greek yogurt* 185 grams
- 1 cup mozzarella 120 grams,shredded
- dash salt
- dash pepper
- ¼ tsp Italian season optional

Directions:

- Preheat oven to 415 °F. Line a large baking sheet with parchment paper.
- In a medium bowl, whisk up eggs. Add Greek yogurt and stir together to a smooth batter. Stir in mozzarella cheese, salt, pepper, and Italian seasoning if desired.
- Pour batter onto your lined baking sheet. With a spoon or spatula, spread batter into a thin oval or rectangle of about 13×11 inches. Bake for 19-21 minutes until golden brown.
- Let flatbread cool down for 5 minutes. Cut into slices or squares for serving. Tastes great with freshly grated parmesan, feta cheese, and/or melted butter.

Beef Jerky

Ingredients:

- Minute steak
- Salt

Directions:

- Preheat airfryer to 175 °F.
- Salt steak and slice into strips.
- Line on airfryer tray ensuring none overlaps
- Cook for 2 hours.

Carnivore Cake

Ingredients:

- 8oz of butter, room temp (I used 8oz of brown butter) you can use salted or unsalted - your choice!
- 8oz of cream cheese (1 brick), room temp
- 8 whole eggs
- You could add vanilla and cinnamon.

Instructions:

- Preheat oven to 350F.
- Combine all ingredients in a high powered blender.
- Blend until well combined. Scrape edges to ensure all ingredients are incorporated.
- Pour into a lined or greased baking dish. (**** ⬚ some people like baking it in a loaf pan to slice and make "French toast". I use a cake

pan so it bakes more quickly and I can enjoy it like a slice of cake lol 🙂)

- Bake at 350F for 25-30min or until a toothpick inserted into the middle comes out clean. *** 🍰 if using a loaf pan, adjust baking time to 40-45min or until the inserted toothpick comes out clean.
- Allow to cool before slicing.
- Serve with fresh whipped cream

Keto

Keto Chicken Salad With A Creamy Dressing

Ingredients:

Chimichurri dressing
- 4 tbsp mayonnaise
- ¼ tbsp red wine vinegar
- ½ cup (¼ oz.) fresh parsley or fresh cilantro
- ½ tbsp red chili peppers, chopped
- 1 tbsp dried oregano
- 1 garlic clove

Chicken thighs
- 1 tbsp olive oil or coconut oil
- 1 lb boneless chicken thighs
- salt and ground black pepper

Serving
- 2 cups (4 oz.) leafy greens
- 1 (7 oz.) avocado, sliced
- ¼ (1 oz.) red onion, sliced

- 1 lemon, cut into wedges (optional)
- ½ red chili pepper, sliced (optional)

Directions:

- Add all the ingredients for the chimichurri dressing to a food processor or a blender. Mix until smooth. Add some water if you prefer a runnier consistency. Set aside.
- Heat a large skillet with olive oil. Season the chicken thighs with salt and pepper. Add them to the hot pan and fry on both sides until completely cooked. It will take about 10-15 minutes depending on the thickness of the meat.
- While the chicken is frying, prepare the vegetables and arrange them on individual plates or a big serving platter. Place the chicken on top and serve with the dressing, a couple of lemon wedges, and chili if you like to add a bit more heat to the dish.

Instant Pot Parmesan Pork With Broccoli

Ingredients:

Parmesan Pork:
- 32 ounce boneless pork shoulder, cut into 3-4 pieces
- 2 ounce Parmesan cheese, grated
- 3/4 cup low-carb tomato sauce, like Rao's brand
- 2 tablespoon unsalted butter
- 1 tablespoon dried basil
- salt and pepper, to taste

Roasted Broccoli:
- 16 ounce broccoli, cut into florets
- 4 tablespoon olive oil
- 1 teaspoon Italian seasoning
- salt and pepper, to taste

Directions:

- Season the pork with salt and pepper, then place into the instant pot
- Add the butter, tomato sauce, parmesan cheese, and dried basil. Stir to incorporate. Seal the instant pot and cook for 50 minutes on the manual setting. Allow the pressure to naturally release (~15 minutes).
- When ~20 minutes is left on the Instant Pot, pre-heat oven to 400F. Place broccoli florets into a baking dish/tray and toss in oil, Italian seasoning, and salt and pepper to taste. Bake for 20-25 minutes or until edges are browned.
-Before serving, shred the pork with 2 forks.

Strawberry Cream Cheese Bites

Ingredients
- 1 cup strawberries(150 g), diced
- 1 teaspoon vanilla extract
- ¼ cup coconut oil(60 g)
- ¾ cup cream cheese(170 g), softened

Directions:
- Place the strawberries in a blender and blend until pureed.
- Add the vanilla extract, coconut oil, and softened cream cheese, and blend until the texture is silky smooth.
- Line a 12-cup muffin with liners (we used silicone liners) or grease with coconut oil. Divide the mixture between the cups.
- Freeze for 2 hours or until solid.
- Store in the freezer.

Keto Coconut Flour Bread

Ingredients:
- ½ cup melted coconut oil, melted (save some for greasing the pan)
- 12 large eggs
- 1 cup (3⅓ oz.) coconut flour

- ½ tsp sea salt
- ½ tsp baking powder

Instructions:
- Preheat the oven to 350°F (175°C). Grease a 9x5x3" (23x13x8cm) loaf pan and set it aside.
- In a large bowl, whisk together the eggs, and coconut oil.
- Add the dry ingredients, and stir until combined.
- Spread the batter in the loaf pan. Bake on the middle rack for 40-50 minutes, or until a toothpick comes out clean, after inserting in the center of the loaf.
- Set aside to cool for 15-20 minutes, and then slice to serve.

Keto Breakfast Fat Bombs

Ingredients:

- 4 hardboiled eggs chopped
- 8 ounces cream cheese see notes for dairy-free options
- 2 tablespoons minced green onion
- 1 lb bacon cooked and crumbled

Instructions:
- In a medium bowl, mix together the chopped hard-boiled eggs, cream cheese, and green onion. Roll into 8 balls. Place the balls in the freezer for 10 minutes to set just a bit.
- Place the crumbled bacon on a plate and roll the balls in the bacon pressing the bacon slightly into the ball. Store in an airtight container in the refrigerator for up to 4 days.

Anti-Inflammatory

Chocolate Overnight Oats

Ingredients:

- 1/2 cup rolled oats
- 1/2 cup non-dairy milk or regular milk
- 1/4 cup non-dairy yogurt or regular yogurt (optional)
- 1 tbsp cocoa or cacao powder
- 1 tbsp maple syrup (or honey, agave, etc)
- 1/2 tbsp chia seeds
- 1/2 tsp vanilla extract
- 1/4 tsp cinnamon
- 1/8 tsp salt

Instructions:

- Add rolled oats, milk, yogurt, cocoa or cacao powder, maple syrup, chia seeds, vanilla extract, cinnamon, and salt to a jar. Mix ingredients together, then seal with a lid.
- Store oats in the refrigerator overnight (or at least 4 hours).
- The next morning (or whenever you are ready to eat), remove the lid and stir the oats. If desired, add a splash of milk to thin the consistency.
- Enjoy the oats directly out of the jar or transfer them to a bowl. Add any toppings of your choosing, like fresh fruit, nut butter, chocolate chips, and granola. Enjoy!

Creamy Chickpea Miso Vegetable Stew

Ingredients:

- 1 tablespoon OLIVE OIL
- 1 large onion, chopped (if tolerated)
- 3 large stalks celery, chopped
- 4 cloves garlic, minced (if tolerated)
- 3 cups cooked chickpeas (2 14.5-ounce cans, drained and rinsed)
- 6 cups vegetable broth

- 1 teaspoon sweet paprika
- 1/4 cup WHITE MISO (you can substitute red or brown miso if that's what you have; use chickpea miso or barley miso if you need the soup to be soy-free)
- 4 carrots, peeled and chopped
- 1 small head cauliflower (~1 lb), cored and cut into bite-sized pieces and florets (4 cups)
- 1 rutabaga, peeled and chopped (substitute 1 turnip, celery root, or Yukon gold potato)
- 1 small bunch kale, washed, stemmed, and chopped
- Salt and pepper as needed

Instructions:

- Add the olive oil to a stockpot over medium heat. When the oil is shimmering, add the onion and celery. Cook for 5-7 minutes, or until the onion isclear and tender.
-Add the garlic and cook for another minute, stirring constantly.
- Add the chickpeas, broth, and paprika to the pot. Bring the broth to a boil, then reduce heat to low. Simmer for 10 minutes, then turn off the heat.
- Place the miso in a small bowl. Use a ladle to transfer a small amount (about 3/4 cup) of broth to to the bowl. Whisk the miso with the broth to create a smooth slurry, then transfer the slurry back to the soup pot. Stir the soup.
- Place about half of the soup into a standing blender and blend till it's totally smooth, then return it to the pot; alternately, you can use an immersion blender to puree half the soup. Stir again.
- Add the carrots, cauliflower, rutabaga, and kale to the pot. Bring the soup back to a low simmer. Simmer for 10-15 minutes, or until all of the vegetables are tender. - Taste the soup and add salt, pepper, and lemon juice as needed. Serve.

Golden Milk Latte

Ingredients:

- 1 cup turmeric powder
- ½ teaspoon ground cloves
- 4 teaspoon ground cinnamon
- 2 teaspoons cardamom powder
- 2 tablespoons ginger powder
- ½-1 tablespoon black pepper (if tolerated)

Directions:
- Add all the ingredients to a container with a lid
-Add the lid and shake it up! And that is it, you have your golden milk latte mix!
- Store it in an airtight container out of direct sunlight. I store mine in my tea cabinet. When you are ready for a latte, mix 1 teaspoon of this mix with your milk of choice. Enjoy!

Corn Chowder

Ingredients:

- 1 Large Onion, chopped (if tolerated)
- 5 1/2 Cups Vegetable broth
- 5 Cups Frozen corn
- 1 Red pepper, chopped (if tolerated)
- 1/8 Tsp Curry powder
- 1/8 Tsp Turmeric
- 1/8 Tsp Cayenne pepper (if tolerated)
- 1/8 Tsp Freshly ground black pepper (if tolerated)

Directions:

- Place 1/2 cup of the vegetable broth in a large pot. - Add the onion and cook, stirring occasionally until onion softens slightly, about 3-4 minutes.

- Add the corn and continue to cook until corn softens slightly about 5 minutes.
- Add 3 cups of the vegetable broth, bring to a boil, reduce heat, cover and cook for about 15 minutes.
- Transfer about half of the corn mixture to a blender and blend until smooth. Return to pan.
- Add the remaining vegetable broth as well as the remaining ingredients.
- Bring back to a boil, reduce heat, cover and simmer for about 10 minutes longer.

Pumpkin Pie

Ingredients:

Base
- 1 cup wholemeal flour
- 1 cup milk of choice

Filling
- 1 can pumpkin puree (15 oz) (I make my own by roasting a whole pumpkin until soft)
- 1 cup milk of choice
- 2 1/2 tsp pure vanilla extract
- 2 tsp cinnamon
- 2 tsp baking powder
- 1 tsp pumpkin pie spice
- 1/2 tsp salt
- 1/3 cup flour, such as spelt, oat,sorghum, or almond
- 1/2 cup maple syrup
- 1 tbsp flaxmeal OR 2 tsp arrowroo
- optional 2 tbsp extra virgin olive oil for richness

Instructions:

- Preheat oven to 400 F, and grease a 10 or 9-inch round pan.

- MIx flour and milk together to form a dough, knead for 5 minutes and then roll out flat.
- Lay base in pie pan
- In a large mixing bowl, whisk all ingredients well. Pour into the pan, and bake 35 minutes. It'll still be gooey after baking.
- Allow to cool completely before transferring uncovered to the fridge to "set" for at least 6 hours before slicing, during which time it will firm up.